CARNIVORE DIET REVOLUTION

Transform Your Life with Meat-Only Nutrition

By

SHARON BYERS

Copyright © 2024 by Sharon Byers

Disclaimer

The information contained in this book is for general informational purposes only. The author and publisher make no representation or warranties of any kind, express or implied, about the completeness, accuracy, reliability, suitability, or availability with respect to the information, products, services, or related graphics contained in this book for any purpose. Any reliance you place on such information is therefore strictly at your own risk.

In no event will the author or publisher be liable for any loss or damage including without limitation, indirect or consequential loss or damage, or any loss or damage whatsoever arising from loss of data or profits arising out of, or in connection with, the use of this book.

While every effort has been made to ensure that the information in this book is accurate and up-to-date, the author and publisher do not warrant that the information will be kept up-to-date, be true, accurate, complete, or non-misleading.

Any views or opinions represented in this book are personal and belong solely to the author and do not represent those of people, institutions, or organizations that the author may or may not be associated with in professional or personal capacity unless explicitly stated.

Table of Contents

INTRODUCTION

The Carnivore Diet Revolution: Why Meat-Only Nutrition Matters

The landscape of dietary advice is a cacophony of conflicting voices. Veganism, paleo, keto, intermittent fasting—each with its proponents, promises, and pitfalls. Yet, amidst this sea of dietary paradigms, one approach is quietly gaining traction, sparking intense debate and fervent support: the carnivore diet. This meat-only diet, at first glance, appears radical, even heretical, in a world increasingly dominated by plant-based nutrition trends. But as more individuals report remarkable health transformations, it's worth exploring why meat-only nutrition might be the revolution we've been waiting for.

Unveiling the Ancestral Wisdom

To understand the carnivore diet, we must journey back in time to the lives of our ancestors. For millions of years, humans thrived as hunter-gatherers, with a significant portion of their diet coming from animal sources. This ancestral way of eating is embedded in our DNA, sculpting our digestive systems and nutritional needs. The idea behind the carnivore diet is to reconnect with this primal heritage, leveraging the foods that fueled human evolution.

Imagine the Paleolithic era, where early humans roamed vast landscapes, hunting mammoths, bison, and deer. These hunts were not just a means of survival but a way of life that provided essential nutrients in their most bioavailable forms. Meat, organs, and fat offered a dense source of calories, vitamins, and minerals necessary for the development of our large brains and robust bodies. This nutrient-dense, satiating diet was pivotal in shaping our physiology.

The Modern Disconnect

Fast forward to the modern age, and our diets have dramatically shifted. The advent of agriculture introduced grains, legumes, and processed foods, while industrialization brought an abundance of sugar-laden and chemically altered products. As our food environment changed, so did our health. Chronic diseases such as obesity, diabetes, and heart disease have surged, raising questions about the role of modern diets in these epidemics.

The carnivore diet challenges this modern dietary paradigm. It posits that many of our health issues stem from a diet incongruent with our evolutionary biology. By eliminating plant-based foods and focusing solely on animal products, proponents argue that we can mitigate inflammation, correct nutrient deficiencies, and restore metabolic health. The notion is not merely to reject modern foods but to embrace a diet that aligns more closely with our genetic heritage.

The Science of Meat-Only Nutrition

At its core, the carnivore diet is grounded in a simple premise: animal foods provide complete nutrition. Unlike plants, which contain anti-nutrients that can interfere with nutrient absorption, animal products are rich in bioavailable vitamins and minerals. For instance, beef liver alone is a powerhouse of essential nutrients, offering high levels of vitamin A, B vitamins, iron, and zinc, among others.

Proteins and fats from animal sources are crucial for numerous bodily functions. Protein, composed of amino acids, is the building block of muscles, tissues, and enzymes. Fat, often vilified in mainstream nutrition, is indispensable for hormone production, brain function, and cellular health. The carnivore diet leverages these macronutrients to promote optimal health, with anecdotal evidence suggesting improvements in energy levels, mental clarity, and physical performance.

Addressing Common Concerns

Understandably, the carnivore diet raises several questions and concerns. Is it safe to exclude all plant foods? What about fiber, antioxidants, and other compounds found in vegetables and fruits? Critics argue that a meat-only diet is extreme and unsustainable in the long term. However, emerging research and personal testimonies paint a more nuanced picture.

Fiber, often touted as essential for digestive health, may not be as crucial as once thought. The carnivore diet advocates claim that the elimination of fibrous plant matter can actually alleviate digestive issues like bloating, constipation, and irritable bowel syndrome (IBS). Instead of relying on fiber, they suggest that a diet rich in fatty meats provides sufficient lubrication for the intestines, while the absence of plant toxins reduces gut inflammation.

Antioxidants, another concern, are indeed vital for combating oxidative stress and inflammation. Yet, animal foods also contain potent antioxidants, such as carnosine and taurine, which are often overlooked. Furthermore, by reducing the intake of inflammatory plant compounds, the body's overall oxidative burden may decrease, reducing the need for high antioxidant intake.

Real-Life Transformations

One of the most compelling aspects of the carnivore diet is the plethora of success stories from individuals who have embraced this unconventional approach. From weight loss and muscle gain to the resolution of chronic conditions like autoimmune diseases, depression, and skin disorders, the testimonies are inspiring.

Take, for example, the case of Mikhaila Peterson, who turned to the carnivore diet after struggling with severe autoimmune disorders for years. Her experience, marked by dramatic improvements in her health and quality of life, has inspired thousands to explore the diet for themselves. Similarly, Dr. Shawn Baker, a prominent advocate of the carnivore diet, has demonstrated through his own athletic performance and patient outcomes that meat-based nutrition can support exceptional health and vitality.

Embracing the Carnivore Revolution

The carnivore diet is not just a fad; it's a revolution grounded in our ancestral past and supported by modern experiences. It challenges us to rethink everything we've been taught about nutrition and to question the role of conventional dietary wisdom in our health crises. While it may not be suitable for everyone, the carnivore diet offers a unique perspective on what it means to nourish our bodies.

As you embark on this journey through "Carnivore Revolution: Transform Your Life with Meat-Only Nutrition," keep an open mind. The following chapters will delve deeper into the scientific underpinnings, practical applications, and transformative potential of a meat-only diet. Whether you're seeking relief from chronic illness, aiming to optimize your performance, or simply curious about the carnivore way, this book will provide the insights and guidance you need.

Why Meat-Only Nutrition Matters

In a world overwhelmed with dietary choices and nutritional advice, the carnivore diet stands out for its simplicity and alignment with human evolution. By focusing on meat, we return to a way of eating that has sustained our species for millennia. This diet isn't just about cutting out plants; it's about rediscovering the nutrient-rich foods that our ancestors thrived on.

The carnivore revolution is more than a diet—it's a movement towards reclaiming our health through natural, unprocessed foods. As you explore the chapters ahead, you'll uncover the power of meat-only nutrition and why it matters in today's health landscape. Welcome to the carnivore revolution—your journey to optimal health starts here.

CHAPTER 1: THE ANCESTRAL DIET

Exploring The Roots Of Human Nutrition

To truly grasp the principles and potential benefits of the carnivore diet, we must delve into the nutritional history of our species. This journey begins with our ancestors, who relied heavily on animal-based foods to survive and thrive. By exploring the roots of human nutrition, we can better understand the physiological and evolutionary foundations that support a meat-centric diet today.

The Paleolithic Era: A Diet Defined by Survival

The Paleolithic era, often referred to as the Old Stone Age, spanned approximately 2.5 million to 10,000 years ago. During this time, early humans, or hominins, were primarily hunter-gatherers. Their diets were dictated by the environment and seasonal availability of food, with a significant emphasis on animal products.

Archaeological evidence reveals that early humans consumed a diverse array of animal foods. Fossilized remains and isotopic analyses of bones show that hominins hunted large game animals such as mammoths, bison, and deer. These hunts were not occasional events but regular and necessary for survival. The ability to procure and process animal meat and fat provided a dense source of calories and nutrients, which were crucial for the development of our large brains and complex social structures.

The Role of Meat in Human Evolution

One of the most significant evolutionary advantages that early humans possessed was the ability to adapt to various environments. This adaptability was, in large part, due to their omnivorous diet, which leaned heavily towards meat consumption. The nutrient density of animal foods played a pivotal role in the evolution of Homo sapiens.

Brain Development

The human brain is an energy-intensive organ, consuming roughly 20% of our daily caloric intake despite comprising only about 2% of our body weight. The development of such a large brain required a reliable and nutrient-dense food source. Meat provided essential nutrients like omega-3 fatty acids, particularly DHA (docosahexaenoic acid), which are vital for brain health and development. The high caloric value of animal fat also supplied the necessary energy to support cognitive functions and neural growth.

Physical Adaptations

Our ancestors exhibited several physical adaptations that facilitated meat consumption. The development of tools for hunting and butchering allowed early humans to effectively procure and process meat. Moreover, the human digestive system evolved to efficiently break down and absorb nutrients from animal products. Unlike herbivores, humans have a relatively short digestive tract, which is well-suited for the digestion of protein and fat-rich foods.

Nutrient Bioavailability

Animal products offer superior bioavailability of essential nutrients compared to plant foods. For instance, heme iron found in meat is more readily absorbed by the body than non-heme iron from plant sources. Similarly, vitamins such as B12, D, and K2 are found predominantly in animal foods. These nutrients are crucial for various bodily functions, including energy production, immune support, and bone health.

The Shift to Agriculture: A Nutritional Turning Point

Around 10,000 years ago, the advent of agriculture marked a significant turning point in human history. The shift from hunting and gathering to farming introduced new dietary staples, such as grains and legumes. This transition, often referred to as the Neolithic Revolution, allowed for the establishment of permanent settlements and the development of civilization. However, it also brought about notable changes in human health and nutrition.

Nutritional Deficiencies

With the reliance on cultivated crops, early agricultural societies experienced a decrease in dietary diversity. Grains became a primary food source, which, while energy-dense, lacked the comprehensive nutrient profile of a meat-based diet. This shift led to the emergence of nutritional deficiencies and related health issues. For instance, skeletal remains from early agricultural communities show signs of iron deficiency anemia, dental caries, and stunted growth, which were less common in hunter-gatherer populations.

Rise in Chronic Diseases

The introduction of grains and legumes also contributed to the rise of chronic diseases. These foods contain anti-nutrients such as lectins, phytates, and gluten, which can interfere with nutrient absorption and cause digestive distress. Additionally, the higher carbohydrate content of a grain-based diet can lead to blood sugar imbalances and increased insulin resistance, paving the way for metabolic disorders like diabetes and obesity.

Reconnecting with Our Nutritional Heritage

In recent years, there has been a growing interest in ancestral diets as a means to combat modern health issues. The carnivore diet, which emphasizes a return to meat-centric eating, draws inspiration from the dietary patterns of our hunter-gatherer ancestors. By prioritizing animal foods and eliminating modern processed products, proponents believe that we can restore metabolic health and overall well-being.

The Benefits of a Meat-Based Diet

A meat-based diet offers numerous health benefits that align with our evolutionary biology. Here are some key advantages:

Nutrient Density

Animal products are rich in essential nutrients, including high-quality protein, healthy fats, vitamins, and minerals. These nutrients are crucial for maintaining muscle mass, supporting immune function, and promoting overall health.

Satiety and Weight Management

Meat is highly satiating, meaning it helps you feel full and satisfied for longer periods. This can lead to reduced calorie intake and easier weight management. Unlike carbohydrate-heavy meals that can cause rapid spikes and crashes in blood sugar levels, protein and fat from animal foods provide steady and sustained energy.

Reduced Inflammation

Chronic inflammation is a common underlying factor in many modern diseases. By eliminating inflammatory plant compounds and focusing on nutrient-dense animal foods, the carnivore diet may help reduce systemic inflammation. Many individuals report improvements in conditions such as arthritis, skin disorders, and autoimmune diseases after adopting a meat-based diet.

Improved Mental Clarity

The brain benefits of a meat-based diet extend beyond its role in evolution. Many people who follow the carnivore diet experience enhanced mental clarity, focus, and mood stability. The high-fat content of animal foods supports brain health, while the absence of sugar and processed carbohydrates helps stabilize blood sugar levels and reduce brain fog.

Personal Testimonials and Scientific Support

The growing body of anecdotal evidence and scientific research supporting the carnivore diet is compelling. Personal testimonials from individuals who have experienced profound health transformations abound. From reversing chronic illnesses to achieving peak physical performance, these stories highlight the potential of a meat-based diet to improve quality of life.

Scientific studies are also beginning to explore the effects of meat-centric nutrition. Research on low-carbohydrate and ketogenic diets, which share similarities with the carnivore diet, has demonstrated benefits such as improved insulin sensitivity, weight loss, and reduced inflammation. As interest in the carnivore diet continues to grow, we can expect more scientific investigation into its health impacts.

Embracing the Ancestral Diet

Adopting the carnivore diet is not about replicating the exact dietary practices of our ancestors. Instead, it's about understanding the principles of ancestral nutrition and applying them in a modern context. This means prioritizing whole, unprocessed animal foods and avoiding the pitfalls of modern dietary habits.

Practical Steps to Get Started

If you're considering the carnivore diet, here are some practical steps to help you get started:

1. Focus on Quality: Choose high-quality, pasture-raised, and grass-fed animal products whenever possible. These sources tend to have better nutrient profiles and are free from added hormones and antibiotics.

2. Prioritize Variety: While beef is a staple in the carnivore diet, incorporating a variety of animal foods can help ensure you get a broad spectrum of nutrients. Include poultry, pork, fish, eggs, and organ meats in your diet.

3. Listen to Your Body: Pay attention to how your body responds to different foods. Some people thrive on a strict carnivore diet, while others may benefit from including small amounts of dairy or seafood. Adjust your diet based on your individual needs and preferences.

4. Stay Hydrated: Adequate hydration is essential, especially when consuming a high-protein diet. Drink plenty of water and consider incorporating bone broth for added electrolytes and minerals.

5. Monitor Your Health: Regularly check in with your healthcare provider to monitor your health markers. Blood tests can help ensure you're meeting your nutritional needs and staying healthy on the carnivore diet.

The Future of Nutrition

As we continue to explore the roots of human nutrition, the carnivore diet offers a unique perspective on how we can optimize our health. By reconnecting with the dietary practices of our ancestors, we may find solutions to many of the health challenges faced by modern society.

The ancestral diet, characterized by a reliance on animal foods, played a crucial role in shaping human evolution. As we face a growing epidemic of chronic diseases and nutritional deficiencies, the carnivore diet provides a compelling case for revisiting our dietary roots. By embracing meat-centric nutrition, we can unlock the potential for improved health, vitality, and well-being. The journey through "Carnivore Revolution: Transform Your Life with Meat-Only Nutrition" continues as we delve deeper into the science, practicalities, and transformative power of the carnivore diet.

CHAPTER 2: THE SCIENCE BEHIND THE CARNIVORE DIET

Understanding the Nutritional Benefits of Meat

As the adage goes, "You are what you eat." This chapter delves into the scientific underpinnings of the carnivore diet, exploring the nutritional benefits of meat and why it stands out as a powerhouse for human health. From macronutrients to micronutrients, we'll uncover how meat fuels our bodies, supports vital functions, and contributes to overall well-being.

The Nutritional Composition of Meat

Meat is an exceptional source of essential nutrients, providing a comprehensive profile of macronutrients and micronutrients necessary for optimal health. Let's break down these components to understand their roles and benefits.

Macronutrients in Meat

Protein: Meat is renowned for its high-quality protein content. Proteins are composed of amino acids, the building blocks of our bodies. They play a crucial role in muscle growth, tissue repair, enzyme production, and hormone regulation. Unlike plant-based proteins, animal proteins contain all nine essential amino acids in ideal ratios, making them complete proteins.

Fats: Meat contains various types of fats, including saturated fats, monounsaturated fats, and polyunsaturated fats. These fats are essential for energy production, cell membrane integrity, hormone synthesis, and the absorption of fat-soluble vitamins (A, D, E, and K). Animal fats, particularly from grass-fed sources, provide beneficial fatty acids like omega-3s, which support brain health and reduce inflammation.

Micronutrients in Meat

Vitamins: Meat is a rich source of several vital vitamins. For instance, vitamin B12, found exclusively in animal products, is crucial for nerve function, red blood cell formation, and DNA synthesis. Meat also supplies significant amounts of vitamins A, D, K2, and various B vitamins, which support metabolic functions, immune health, and more.

Minerals: Meat provides a range of essential minerals, including iron, zinc, selenium, and phosphorus. Heme iron, the type of iron found in meat, is more easily absorbed by the body compared to non-heme iron from plant sources. This makes meat an important dietary component for preventing iron-deficiency anemia. Zinc is vital for immune function, wound healing, and DNA synthesis, while selenium acts as an antioxidant and supports thyroid health.

Bioavailability: The Advantage of Animal Foods

One of the key advantages of meat is the bioavailability of its nutrients. Bioavailability refers to the proportion of nutrients that can be absorbed and utilized by the body. Animal foods typically offer superior bioavailability compared to plant foods due to the absence of anti-nutrients like phytates, oxalates, and lectins that can inhibit nutrient absorption.

For example, the heme iron in meat is absorbed at a rate of 15-35%, whereas non-heme iron from plants is absorbed at a rate of only 2-20%. Similarly, the vitamin A in animal foods (retinol) is more readily used by the body compared to the beta-carotene found in plants, which must be converted to retinol before it can be utilized.

Meat and Metabolism

The macronutrient composition of meat supports efficient metabolism and energy production. Here's how:

Protein and Thermogenesis: Protein has a high thermic effect, meaning it requires more energy to digest, absorb, and process compared to fats and carbohydrates. This thermogenic effect boosts metabolism, aiding in weight management and fat loss. Additionally, protein helps maintain muscle mass, which is critical for a healthy metabolism.

Fat and Energy: Dietary fats are a dense source of energy, providing 9 calories per gram compared to 4 calories per gram from protein and carbohydrates. The fats in meat, particularly saturated fats, are readily used by the body for sustained energy, supporting physical performance and cognitive function.

The Role of Cholesterol and Saturated Fat

Cholesterol and saturated fat have long been demonized in mainstream nutrition, but recent research is challenging these notions. Cholesterol is a vital molecule involved in hormone production, cell membrane integrity, and brain function. The body tightly regulates cholesterol levels, producing it as needed regardless of dietary intake.

Saturated fat, found abundantly in meat, plays several important roles, including the production of hormones such as testosterone, the absorption of fat-soluble vitamins, and providing a stable source of energy. Studies have shown that dietary saturated fat does not correlate strongly with an increased risk of heart disease, contrary to popular belief.

The Inflammatory Response

A primary criticism of meat consumption is its purported link to inflammation. However, inflammation in the context of a balanced diet is not inherently negative; it is a natural and necessary response to injury and infection. Chronic inflammation, on the other hand, is problematic and linked to various diseases.

Meat, particularly from grass-fed and pasture-raised animals, contains anti-inflammatory nutrients such as omega-3 fatty acids and conjugated linoleic acid (CLA). These compounds help modulate the inflammatory response and support overall health. Furthermore, by eliminating processed foods and inflammatory plant compounds, the carnivore diet may help reduce chronic inflammation.

The Gut Microbiome and Meat Consumption

The gut microbiome, composed of trillions of microorganisms, plays a crucial role in digestion, immune function, and overall health. Diet significantly influences the composition and function of the gut microbiome. While fiber from plant foods is often emphasized for gut health, the carnivore diet offers a different perspective.

Gut Health on a Carnivore Diet: Many individuals report improvements in digestive health, including relief from bloating, gas, and irritable bowel syndrome (IBS) symptoms, after adopting the carnivore diet. This can be attributed to the elimination of fiber and anti-nutrients that can irritate the gut lining and disrupt microbiome balance.

Short-Chain Fatty Acids (SCFAs): SCFAs, such as butyrate, are produced by the fermentation of fiber in the colon and are beneficial for gut health. While the carnivore diet lacks fiber, it doesn't necessarily lead to a deficiency in SCFAs. Ketones, produced during fat metabolism in a low-carb, high-fat diet, can serve as an alternative fuel source for gut cells, potentially mimicking the effects of SCFAs.

Carnivore Diet and Chronic Diseases

Emerging evidence suggests that the carnivore diet may offer benefits for various chronic diseases. Here's a closer look at how meat-centric nutrition can impact some common conditions:

Obesity and Metabolic Syndrome: The high protein content of the carnivore diet promotes satiety and reduces overall calorie intake, aiding in weight loss. Additionally, the low-carbohydrate nature of the diet helps stabilize blood sugar levels and improve insulin sensitivity, which are critical factors in managing metabolic syndrome and type 2 diabetes.

Cardiovascular Health: Contrary to popular belief, meat consumption does not necessarily increase the risk of heart disease. A diet rich in animal fats can improve lipid profiles by increasing HDL (good) cholesterol and reducing triglycerides. Furthermore, the anti-inflammatory effects of omega-3s and CLA in meat contribute to cardiovascular health.

Autoimmune Diseases: Many individuals with autoimmune conditions report significant improvements on the carnivore diet. By eliminating potential dietary triggers, such as gluten and lectins, and providing anti-inflammatory nutrients, the diet may help modulate the immune system and reduce autoimmune flare-ups.

Mental Health: The brain requires a constant supply of high-quality nutrients to function optimally. The carnivore diet provides essential nutrients like omega-3s, B vitamins, and minerals that support cognitive health. Anecdotal reports suggest that this diet can improve mood, reduce anxiety, and enhance mental clarity.

Practical Considerations and Potential Challenges

While the carnivore diet offers numerous benefits, it's essential to consider practical aspects and potential challenges:

Nutrient Balance: Ensuring a balanced intake of various animal foods is crucial to avoid nutrient deficiencies. Incorporating a variety of meats, fish, eggs, and organ meats can help achieve a comprehensive nutrient profile.

Electrolyte Management: The carnivore diet can lead to increased water and electrolyte excretion, especially during the initial adaptation phase. Consuming adequate salt and staying hydrated are essential to prevent imbalances and support overall health.

Social and Cultural Factors: Adopting a meat-only diet can present social and cultural challenges. Dining out, attending social events, and navigating family meals may require careful planning and communication to maintain dietary adherence.

The Science Supports Meat-Based Nutrition

The scientific evidence supporting the nutritional benefits of meat is robust and compelling. From macronutrients to micronutrients, meat provides a complete and bioavailable source of essential nutrients that support optimal health. The carnivore diet, rooted in our evolutionary history, offers a practical and effective approach to addressing modern health challenges.

As you continue your journey through "Carnivore Revolution: Transform Your Life with Meat-Only Nutrition," keep in mind the scientific principles that underscore the diet's potential. Understanding the nutritional benefits of meat empowers you to make informed decisions about your health and well-being. The next chapters will delve deeper into practical applications, meal planning, and the transformative power of the carnivore diet.

CHAPTER 3: GETTING STARTED

Transitioning to a Meat-Only Lifestyle

Embarking on the carnivore diet may seem daunting, especially if you're accustomed to a diet rich in plant-based foods and carbohydrates. However, transitioning to a meat-only lifestyle can be a smooth and rewarding process with the right guidance and mindset. This chapter will provide you with practical tips, strategies, and insights to help you successfully adopt and thrive on the carnivore diet.

Understanding the Basics

Before diving into the practical steps, it's essential to understand the fundamental principles of the carnivore diet. At its core, the diet involves consuming only animal-based foods and eliminating all plant-based foods and processed products. This includes all meats (beef, pork, poultry, fish), animal fats, eggs, and dairy (for those who tolerate it). The goal is to simplify your diet to nutrient-dense, bioavailable foods that promote optimal health.

Step 1: Preparing for the Transition

Mindset and Motivation: Success on the carnivore diet begins with a clear understanding of your reasons for making the switch. Whether it's for health improvements, weight loss, mental clarity, or curiosity, having a strong motivation will help you stay committed. Educate yourself about the benefits and challenges of the diet to set realistic expectations.

Gradual vs. Cold Turkey: Decide whether you want to transition gradually or go "cold turkey." A gradual transition involves slowly reducing plant foods and increasing animal foods over a few weeks. This approach can help your body adjust more comfortably. Going cold turkey means making the switch all at once, which can lead to a faster adaptation period but may also come with more pronounced initial symptoms.

Step 2: Stocking Your Kitchen

Quality Over Quantity: Focus on sourcing high-quality animal products. Whenever possible, choose grass-fed, pasture-raised, and wild-caught options. These sources provide better nutrient profiles and fewer toxins than conventionally raised animals.

Variety is Key: While beef is a staple in the carnivore diet, incorporating a variety of animal foods ensures you get a broad spectrum of nutrients. Stock your kitchen with different cuts of beef, pork, poultry, fish, eggs, and organ meats. Organ meats like liver, heart, and kidneys are exceptionally nutrient-dense and should be included regularly.

Essential Kitchen Tools: Equip your kitchen with tools that make meal preparation easier and more enjoyable. A good set of knives, a cast-iron skillet, a slow cooker, and an air fryer can simplify cooking and expand your culinary options.

Step 3: Planning Your Meals

Simple and Satisfying: The carnivore diet doesn't require elaborate recipes or meal plans. Keep it simple with basic cooking methods like grilling, baking, broiling, and slow cooking. Focus on preparing satisfying meals that highlight the natural flavors of the meat.

Sample Meal Ideas:
- Breakfast: Scrambled eggs cooked in butter, bacon, or a steak
- Lunch: Grilled chicken thighs, burger patties, or salmon fillets
- Dinner: Ribeye steak, pork chops, or lamb chops
- Snacks: Hard-boiled eggs, beef jerky (without added sugars), or cheese (if tolerated)

Organizing Your Week: Plan your meals for the week to streamline grocery shopping and meal preparation. Batch cooking and meal prepping can save time and ensure you have carnivore-friendly meals ready when hunger strikes.

Step 4: Navigating the Transition Phase

Adapting to Change: Your body may take time to adjust to the carnivore diet, especially if you're coming from a high-carb or plant-based diet. It's common to experience temporary symptoms such as fatigue, headaches, and digestive changes as your body adapts to burning fat for fuel.

Electrolyte Management: One of the most crucial aspects of transitioning is maintaining proper electrolyte balance. As you reduce carbohydrate intake, your body excretes more water and electrolytes, which can lead to imbalances. Ensure you consume adequate salt, potassium, and magnesium to support hydration and prevent symptoms like muscle cramps and fatigue.

Listening to Your Body: Pay attention to how your body responds and adjust accordingly. Some people may experience initial cravings for carbohydrates or sweets, which often diminish as your body adapts. Staying hydrated, getting enough rest, and managing stress can help ease the transition.

Step 5: Long-Term Sustainability

Customizing Your Diet: The carnivore diet is flexible and can be tailored to individual needs and preferences. While some people thrive on a strict meat-only diet, others may find they do well with the inclusion of certain dairy products or seafood. Experiment and find what works best for you.

Social Situations: Navigating social events and dining out can be challenging. Plan ahead by checking menus, bringing your own food, or eating before attending events. Communicate your dietary choices with friends and family to seek their support and understanding.

Monitoring Your Health: Regularly check in with your healthcare provider to monitor your health markers. Blood tests can help ensure you're meeting your nutritional needs and maintaining overall health. Track your progress, noting any changes in energy levels, mental clarity, and physical well-being.

Common Challenges and Solutions

Dealing with Criticism: The carnivore diet may attract skepticism or criticism from others. Arm yourself with knowledge and be prepared to explain your reasons for choosing this lifestyle. Focus on your personal experiences and the positive changes you've noticed.

Digestive Adjustments: Some people may experience changes in digestion, such as constipation or diarrhea, during the transition. Ensuring adequate hydration, consuming enough fat, and including organ meats can help alleviate these issues. If problems persist, consider seeking advice from a healthcare professional or a carnivore diet community.

Boredom and Variety: Eating the same foods repeatedly can lead to boredom. Experiment with different cuts of meat, cooking methods, and seasonings to keep your meals interesting. Explore recipes that incorporate various animal products to expand your culinary repertoire.

Success Stories and Inspiration

Hearing from others who have successfully transitioned to the carnivore diet can be motivating and reassuring. Here are a few inspiring success stories:

Kelly's Journey: Kelly struggled with chronic fatigue and autoimmune issues for years. After transitioning to the carnivore diet, she experienced increased energy levels, reduced inflammation, and a significant improvement in her overall health. Kelly now shares her journey on social media, inspiring others to explore the benefits of meat-based nutrition.

John's Transformation: John battled obesity and metabolic syndrome for most of his adult life. Skeptical but desperate for change, he decided to try the carnivore diet. Within months, John lost over 50 pounds, reversed his insulin resistance, and regained his vitality. His transformation story has encouraged many others to reconsider their dietary choices.

Lisa's Mental Clarity: Lisa, a busy professional, noticed a decline in her cognitive function and productivity. Seeking a solution, she adopted the carnivore diet and was amazed by the results. Her mental clarity, focus, and mood significantly improved, allowing her to excel in her career and personal life.

Embrace the Carnivore Lifestyle

Transitioning to a meat-only lifestyle is a journey that requires preparation, dedication, and an open mind. By understanding the basics, planning your meals, and navigating the transition phase, you can set yourself up for success. Remember to listen to your body, customize the diet to your needs, and seek support from like-minded individuals.

The carnivore diet is more than just a way of eating; it's a transformative approach to health that reconnects us with our ancestral roots. As you embark on this journey, embrace the simplicity, nutrient density, and potential benefits of a meat-centric lifestyle. The subsequent chapters will delve deeper into the intricacies of the diet, offering practical tips, scientific insights, and inspirational stories to guide you along the way.

Welcome to the carnivore revolution—your path to optimal health and vitality starts here.

CHAPTER 4: MACRONUTRIENTS AND MICRONUTRIENTS IN MEAT

Comprehensive Guide to Nutrient Intake

Meat is more than just a source of protein; it's a nutrient powerhouse packed with essential macronutrients and micronutrients that fuel our bodies and support overall health. This chapter provides a comprehensive guide to the nutrient intake from meat, highlighting the crucial roles each nutrient plays and how the carnivore diet ensures you get everything you need to thrive.

Macronutrients in Meat

Protein: The Building Block of Life

Protein is perhaps the most celebrated macronutrient in meat, and for good reason. It is essential for building and repairing tissues, producing enzymes and hormones, and supporting overall bodily functions. Here's a closer look at why protein is vital:

- Complete Protein: Meat contains all nine essential amino acids that our bodies cannot produce on their own. This makes it a complete protein source, crucial for muscle repair, immune function, and the production of neurotransmitters.

- Muscle Maintenance and Growth: Adequate protein intake is necessary for maintaining and building muscle mass. This is especially important for athletes, older adults, and anyone looking to improve their physical performance.

- Satiety and Weight Management: Protein is highly satiating, meaning it helps you feel full and satisfied, reducing the likelihood of overeating. This can be beneficial for weight management and controlling appetite.

Fats: Essential Energy and More

Fats are a dense source of energy and play a myriad of roles in maintaining health. Meat provides various types of fats, each with unique benefits:

- Saturated Fats: Found predominantly in red meat and animal products, saturated fats are essential for hormone production, brain health, and cell membrane integrity. Despite past misconceptions, recent studies have shown that saturated fats are not directly linked to heart disease when consumed as part of a balanced diet.

- Monounsaturated Fats: These healthy fats are abundant in meats like pork and are known for their heart-protective properties. They help reduce bad cholesterol levels and are beneficial for cardiovascular health.

- Polyunsaturated Fats: These include omega-3 and omega-6 fatty acids. Omega-3s, in particular, are found in fatty fish and are known for their anti-inflammatory properties, supporting brain health and reducing the risk of chronic diseases.

The Importance of Cholesterol

Cholesterol, often misunderstood, is a vital component of every cell in the body. It is involved in producing hormones, vitamin D, and bile acids necessary for fat digestion. While the body can produce cholesterol, dietary cholesterol from meat plays a role in maintaining optimal levels for various bodily functions.

Micronutrients in Meat

Meat is an excellent source of essential vitamins and minerals, each playing a unique role in maintaining health and preventing deficiencies.

Vitamins: The Vital Catalysts

- Vitamin B12: Found exclusively in animal products, vitamin B12 is crucial for red blood cell formation, nerve function, and DNA synthesis. Deficiency can lead to anemia, neurological issues, and cognitive impairments.

- Vitamin A: Present in liver and other organ meats, vitamin A supports vision, immune function, and skin health. Unlike beta-carotene from plants, the retinol form in meat is readily usable by the body.

- Vitamin D: Fatty fish and liver are rich sources of vitamin D, essential for bone health, immune function, and mood regulation. It helps in the absorption of calcium and phosphorus, critical for maintaining healthy bones and teeth.

- B Vitamins (B1, B2, B3, B5, B6): These vitamins are abundant in meat and play pivotal roles in energy production, brain function, and cell metabolism. They support the conversion of food into energy and are necessary for healthy skin, eyes, and liver.

Minerals: The Essential Elements

- Iron: Meat provides heme iron, which is more easily absorbed by the body than non-heme iron from plant sources. Iron is vital for transporting oxygen in the blood, supporting energy levels, and preventing anemia.

- Zinc: This mineral is important for immune function, wound healing, and DNA synthesis. It also supports growth and development, making it crucial for children and pregnant women.

- Selenium: Found in high amounts in organ meats, selenium acts as a powerful antioxidant, protecting cells from damage and supporting thyroid health.

- Phosphorus: This mineral is essential for bone health, energy production, and maintaining the body's acid-base balance. Meat is an excellent source of bioavailable phosphorus.

Bioavailability: The Key Advantage of Meat

Bioavailability refers to the proportion of nutrients that can be absorbed and utilized by the body. Meat offers superior bioavailability of nutrients compared to plant-based foods. Here's why:

- Heme Iron: The heme iron in meat is absorbed at a rate of 15-35%, whereas non-heme iron from plants is absorbed at a rate of only 2-20%. This makes meat a crucial dietary component for preventing iron-deficiency anemia.

- Vitamin A: The retinol form of vitamin A found in animal products is more readily absorbed and utilized by the body compared to beta-carotene from plant sources, which must be converted to retinol.

- Complete Proteins: The amino acid profile of animal proteins matches our own needs more closely than plant proteins, ensuring that all essential amino acids are available in the right proportions for bodily functions.

Practical Tips for Maximizing Nutrient Intake

Incorporating Variety: While muscle meats like steak and chicken are popular, incorporating a variety of animal foods ensures you get a broad spectrum of nutrients. Organ meats, seafood, eggs, and dairy (if tolerated) can provide additional vitamins and minerals.

Cooking Methods: How you cook your meat can affect nutrient retention. Methods like grilling, broiling, and slow cooking preserve more nutrients compared to high-heat frying or prolonged boiling. Avoid overcooking to retain the maximum nutritional value.

Balancing Fats: Include a mix of fatty and lean cuts to balance your intake of different types of fats. For instance, pair lean meats like chicken breast with fatty cuts like ribeye steak or pork belly to ensure a good balance of saturated and unsaturated fats.

Addressing Common Concerns

Nutrient Deficiencies: One concern about the carnivore diet is the potential for nutrient deficiencies. However, a well-planned carnivore diet that includes a variety of meats, organ meats, and seafood can provide all essential nutrients. Regular monitoring of health markers through blood tests can help identify and address any deficiencies early on.

Calcium Intake: While meat itself is not a significant source of calcium, incorporating bone broth and dairy products (if tolerated) can help meet your calcium needs. Additionally, the high bioavailability of other minerals like phosphorus and vitamin D in meat supports bone health.

Fiber and Gut Health: The carnivore diet eliminates dietary fiber, which can raise concerns about gut health. However, many people report improvements in digestive issues on this diet. Animal foods are highly digestible and do not contain anti-nutrients found in plant foods that can irritate the gut. Ensuring adequate hydration and electrolyte balance can support digestive health.

Real-Life Nutrient Profiles

Beef Liver: Often considered a superfood, beef liver is rich in vitamin A, B vitamins, iron, and selenium. A small serving can provide a significant portion of your daily nutrient needs.

Salmon: This fatty fish is an excellent source of omega-3 fatty acids, vitamin D, and high-quality protein. Regular consumption supports heart and brain health.

Eggs: Eggs are a versatile and nutrient-dense food, providing high-quality protein, vitamin B12, vitamin D, and choline, essential for brain health.

Pork: Pork offers a good mix of monounsaturated fats, complete proteins, and B vitamins. Including various cuts, from tenderloin to pork belly, ensures a balanced intake of nutrients.

Embrace Nutrient-Dense Eating

Understanding the macronutrient and micronutrient composition of meat highlights why the carnivore diet can be incredibly nourishing. By focusing on a variety of high-quality animal foods and mindful preparation methods, you can ensure a comprehensive nutrient intake that supports overall health and well-being.

As you continue your journey with the carnivore diet, remember that quality, variety, and bioavailability are key to reaping the full benefits. The next chapter will guide you through practical meal planning and preparation tips to make the most of your meat-based lifestyle. Embrace the nutrient density of meat and enjoy the myriad benefits it offers for your health.

CHAPTER 5: HEALTH BENEFITS OF THE CARNIVORE DIET

From Weight Loss to Mental Clarity

The carnivore diet, rooted in our ancestral eating habits, offers a range of health benefits that extend beyond the simplicity of its food choices. By focusing solely on nutrient-dense animal products, many people have experienced significant improvements in their physical and mental well-being. This chapter explores the various health benefits of the carnivore diet, from weight loss to enhanced mental clarity, backed by scientific insights and real-life success stories.

Weight Loss and Body Composition

Satiety and Appetite Control

One of the most compelling benefits of the carnivore diet is its impact on appetite regulation and satiety. Animal proteins and fats are highly satiating, meaning they help you feel full and satisfied for longer periods. This can lead to a natural reduction in calorie intake without the need for conscious restriction. Key factors include:

- Protein's Role: Protein is known to stimulate the release of hormones like peptide YY and GLP-1, which signal fullness and reduce hunger.
- Fat Metabolism: Dietary fat slows the digestion process, keeping you feeling satisfied and preventing overeating.

Enhanced Fat Loss

By eliminating carbohydrates, the carnivore diet shifts the body's primary fuel source from glucose to fats. This metabolic state, known as ketosis, promotes efficient fat burning and can lead to significant weight loss. Benefits of ketosis include:

- Increased Fat Oxidation: With reduced insulin levels and an increase in fat oxidation, the body becomes more adept at utilizing stored fat for energy.
- Reduced Insulin Resistance: Lower carbohydrate intake helps decrease insulin resistance, which is often associated with obesity and metabolic syndrome.

Muscle Preservation

Despite being in a calorie deficit, the high protein content of the carnivore diet supports muscle preservation and growth. Protein provides the necessary building blocks for muscle repair and maintenance, which is crucial during weight loss to ensure that the weight lost comes predominantly from fat rather than muscle tissue.

Improved Mental Clarity and Cognitive Function

Brain Fuel

The brain thrives on ketones, which are produced during the metabolism of fats. Ketones provide a stable and efficient source of energy for the brain, leading to enhanced cognitive function. Many people report experiencing improved mental clarity, focus, and memory on the carnivore diet.

Reduced Brain Fog

Chronic brain fog can be debilitating, affecting productivity and quality of life. The carnivore diet eliminates potential dietary culprits like sugar, gluten, and other inflammatory plant compounds that can contribute to brain fog. The result is a clearer, more focused mind.

Mood Stabilization

Mood swings and anxiety can be linked to fluctuations in blood sugar levels. By stabilizing blood sugar and providing a steady source of fuel, the carnivore diet can help reduce mood swings and promote emotional stability. Additionally, the anti-inflammatory properties of a meat-based diet can alleviate symptoms of depression and anxiety.

Enhanced Physical Performance

Increased Energy Levels

Many people transitioning to the carnivore diet report a significant increase in energy levels. By relying on fat for fuel, which provides a more consistent and sustained energy source than carbohydrates, you can avoid the energy crashes associated with carb-heavy meals.

Improved Endurance

Endurance athletes have started to explore the benefits of a low-carb, high-fat diet. The carnivore diet enhances the body's ability to utilize fat for prolonged energy, which can improve endurance performance. The reduction in muscle glycogen depletion and the ability to tap into abundant fat stores helps sustain energy levels during long periods of physical activity.

Enhanced Recovery

The high protein intake from the carnivore diet aids in muscle repair and recovery. Additionally, the anti-inflammatory effects of a meat-based diet can reduce muscle soreness and speed up recovery times after intense workouts.

Hormonal Balance

Insulin Regulation

As mentioned earlier, the carnivore diet can significantly improve insulin sensitivity. By reducing carbohydrate intake, insulin levels stabilize, reducing the risk of insulin resistance, which is a precursor to type 2 diabetes.

Leptin Sensitivity

Leptin is a hormone that regulates hunger and energy balance. Improved leptin sensitivity on the carnivore diet helps your body better regulate fat storage and hunger signals, contributing to weight loss and maintenance.

Sex Hormones

Balanced intake of dietary fats is crucial for the production of sex hormones like testosterone and estrogen. The carnivore diet's emphasis on healthy animal fats supports hormonal health and can improve issues related to hormonal imbalances, such as low libido and menstrual irregularities.

Gut Health and Digestion

Simplified Digestion

Meat is highly digestible and free from anti-nutrients found in plant-based foods, such as lectins, oxalates, and phytates, which can interfere with nutrient absorption and irritate the gut. The carnivore diet simplifies digestion and can alleviate symptoms of irritable bowel syndrome (IBS), bloating, and other digestive issues.

Healing the Gut

For individuals with gut disorders like Crohn's disease, ulcerative colitis, or leaky gut syndrome, the carnivore diet can be therapeutic. By eliminating inflammatory foods and focusing on nutrient-dense animal products, the gut lining has the opportunity to heal and regenerate.

Microbiome Balance

Contrary to common belief, the carnivore diet can support a healthy gut microbiome. By reducing the intake of fermentable fibers that feed harmful bacteria and focusing on easily digestible animal proteins, the diet promotes a balanced microbiome and reduces gut inflammation.

Skin Health

Reduction in Acne

Many people report significant improvements in skin conditions like acne after adopting the carnivore diet. Removing processed foods, sugars, and inflammatory plant compounds helps reduce acne outbreaks. The diet's anti-inflammatory properties also play a role in skin health.

Anti-Aging Benefits

The high nutrient density of the carnivore diet, including vitamins A, E, and D, supports skin health and reduces signs of aging. These nutrients promote collagen production, skin elasticity, and repair, contributing to a youthful appearance.

Autoimmune Disease Management

Reduced Inflammation

Chronic inflammation is a common driver of autoimmune diseases. The carnivore diet's focus on anti-inflammatory foods can help reduce systemic inflammation, alleviating symptoms of conditions like rheumatoid arthritis, lupus, and multiple sclerosis.

Symptom Improvement

Many individuals with autoimmune diseases report a significant reduction in symptoms when following the carnivore diet. By eliminating potential triggers found in plant foods and processed products, the body can achieve a state of reduced immune system activation and better symptom control.

Cardiovascular Health

Cholesterol Management

While conventional wisdom has linked meat consumption with high cholesterol, recent research suggests that dietary cholesterol and saturated fat from high-quality animal products do not necessarily increase the risk of heart disease. The carnivore diet can improve lipid profiles by increasing HDL (good cholesterol) and reducing triglycerides.

Blood Pressure Regulation

By reducing carbohydrate intake and improving insulin sensitivity, the carnivore diet can help regulate blood pressure. Additionally, the reduction in inflammation and improved electrolyte balance contribute to cardiovascular health.

Real-Life Success Stories

Sarah's Transformation

Sarah struggled with obesity, type 2 diabetes, and chronic fatigue. After transitioning to the carnivore diet, she lost over 80 pounds, reversed her diabetes, and regained her energy. Her mental clarity and mood improved significantly, transforming her outlook on life.

Mike's Recovery

Mike suffered from severe digestive issues and inflammatory bowel disease. The carnivore diet provided relief from his symptoms, allowing his gut to heal. He experienced improved digestion, reduced inflammation, and a newfound sense of well-being.

Laura's Mental Health

Laura battled with depression and anxiety for years. After adopting the carnivore diet, she noticed a dramatic improvement in her mood and mental clarity. Her anxiety diminished, and she felt more balanced and in control of her emotions.

Embrace the Benefits

The health benefits of the carnivore diet extend across various aspects of physical and mental well-being. From weight loss and improved body composition to enhanced cognitive function and better digestion, the diet offers a transformative approach to nutrition. By focusing on nutrient-dense, bioavailable animal products, you can experience profound changes in your health and vitality.

As you continue exploring the carnivore lifestyle, remember that individual experiences may vary. Listen to your body, customize the diet to your needs, and consult with healthcare professionals as needed. The next chapter will delve into practical meal planning and preparation tips to help you make the most of your carnivore journey. Embrace the benefits and thrive on the path to optimal health.

CHAPTER 6: COMMON MISCONCEPTIONS

Debunking Myths And Addressing Concerns

The carnivore diet, despite its growing popularity and numerous success stories, is often met with skepticism and misconceptions. In this chapter, we'll address common myths surrounding the carnivore diet and provide evidence-based insights to clarify misunderstandings. By debunking these myths and addressing concerns, you'll gain a clearer understanding of the diet's principles and potential benefits.

Myth 1: Lack of Nutrient Diversity

Reality: While the carnivore diet eliminates plant-based foods, it emphasizes nutrient-dense animal products that provide a wide array of essential nutrients. Meat, organs, and seafood offer high-quality proteins, healthy fats, vitamins, and minerals necessary for optimal health. Variability in cuts, types of meat, and cooking methods ensures nutrient diversity.

Myth 2: Nutrient Deficiencies

Reality: Contrary to belief, a well-planned carnivore diet can meet all essential nutrient requirements. Meat is rich in bioavailable nutrients like iron, vitamin B12, zinc, and omega-3 fatty acids. Including organ meats and seafood further enhances nutrient intake. Regular monitoring and supplementation, if necessary, can mitigate any potential deficiencies.

Myth 3: Increased Risk of Heart Disease

Reality: Recent research challenges the association between saturated fat intake from animal products and heart disease. The carnivore diet may improve lipid profiles by increasing HDL (good cholesterol) and reducing triglycerides. It focuses on high-quality fats from sources like grass-fed beef and fatty fish, which are beneficial for cardiovascular health.

Myth 4: Lack of Fiber

Reality: While the carnivore diet excludes fiber-rich plant foods, it does not necessarily lead to fiber deficiency. Meat is highly digestible, requiring less digestive effort and reducing gastrointestinal distress. The diet supports gut health by eliminating anti-nutrients and inflammatory compounds found in some plant foods.

Myth 5: Impact on Gut Microbiome

Reality: Contrary to concerns, the carnivore diet can promote a healthy gut microbiome by reducing fermentable fibers that feed harmful bacteria. Animal proteins and fats are easily digestible and do not contribute to gut inflammation. Many individuals report improvements in digestive issues, such as bloating and irritable bowel syndrome (IBS).

Myth 6: Sustainability and Ethical Concerns

Reality: While ethical considerations vary among individuals, the carnivore diet can be sustainable when sourcing from responsible and humane practices. Regenerative agriculture and ethical farming practices support animal welfare and environmental stewardship. Personal ethics and dietary choices can align with sustainable and health-conscious principles.

Myth 7: Long-Term Health Risks

Reality: Long-term studies on the carnivore diet are limited, making it challenging to assess extended health impacts definitively. However, short-term studies and anecdotal evidence suggest potential benefits, including weight loss, improved metabolic health, and enhanced well-being. Individual health outcomes may vary based on genetic predispositions and lifestyle factors.

Addressing Concerns

Variety and Sustainability: Incorporating a variety of animal products ensures nutrient diversity and supports environmental sustainability. Choose grass-fed beef, pasture-raised poultry, wild-caught fish, and organ meats for optimal nutrient intake and ethical considerations.

Monitoring Health Markers: Regularly monitor health markers, including blood lipids, nutrient levels, and overall well-being, to assess the impact of the carnivore diet on your health. Consult healthcare professionals to address any concerns or adjustments needed.

Personalization and Flexibility: The carnivore diet can be personalized to individual preferences and health goals. Some individuals may benefit from occasional inclusion of dairy or seafood, depending on tolerances and nutritional needs. Flexibility allows for adaptation based on lifestyle factors and health outcomes.

Embrace Clarity and Understanding

By debunking common myths and addressing concerns surrounding the carnivore diet, you gain clarity on its principles and potential benefits. Understanding the nutrient density, metabolic advantages, and sustainability aspects helps navigate dietary choices effectively. As you explore the carnivore lifestyle, prioritize informed decisions, personal health assessments, and ongoing education to optimize your well-being.

The subsequent chapters will delve deeper into practical strategies for meal planning, nutrient optimization, and long-term sustainability on the carnivore diet. Embrace clarity, challenge misconceptions, and thrive on the path to optimal health and vitality with a well-informed approach.

CHAPTER 7: CARNIVORE DIET AND GUT HEALTH

Improving Digestion and Reducing Inflammation

The relationship between diet and gut health is profound, influencing overall well-being and immune function. The carnivore diet, centered around animal products, presents a unique perspective on gut health by eliminating potentially irritating plant compounds and focusing on nutrient-dense, easily digestible foods. In this chapter, we explore how the carnivore diet can positively impact digestion, reduce inflammation, and promote gut health.

Simplified Digestion Process

High Digestibility

Meat, particularly muscle meats, is highly digestible compared to plant-based foods that may contain fiber and anti-nutrients. The absence of complex carbohydrates and plant fibers in the carnivore diet simplifies the digestive process, reducing the workload on the gut and minimizing gastrointestinal distress.

Reduced Gut Irritants

Plants contain compounds like lectins, phytates, and oxalates, which can irritate the gut lining and interfere with nutrient absorption. By excluding these substances, the carnivore diet removes potential triggers for digestive issues such as bloating, gas, and discomfort.

Improvement in Digestive Disorders

Many individuals with chronic digestive disorders, including irritable bowel syndrome (IBS) and inflammatory bowel disease (IBD), report significant improvements on the carnivore diet. By eliminating problematic foods and focusing on nutrient-dense animal products, the diet allows the gut to heal and function optimally.

Gut Microbiome Balance

Impact on Microbial Diversity

Contrary to concerns, the carnivore diet can support a healthy gut microbiome by promoting a balanced environment. While plant-based diets often emphasize fiber for gut health, animal products provide essential nutrients and amino acids that support microbial diversity and metabolic functions.

Reduction in Inflammatory Response

Chronic inflammation in the gut can lead to digestive disorders and systemic health issues. The carnivore diet's focus on anti-inflammatory foods, such as fatty fish and grass-fed meats, helps reduce gut inflammation and supports overall immune function.

Adaptation Period

Transitioning to the carnivore diet may involve an adaptation period for the gut microbiome. Initial changes in gut flora composition may occur as the digestive system adjusts to a different dietary approach. Individuals may experience temporary digestive discomfort during this phase, known as the "adaptation period."

Nutrient Absorption and Utilization

Enhanced Nutrient Bioavailability

Meat is rich in bioavailable nutrients such as heme iron, vitamin B12, and zinc, which are essential for energy production, immune function, and overall health. The high bioavailability of nutrients in animal products ensures efficient absorption and utilization by the body, supporting optimal nutrient status.

Vitamin and Mineral Density

Organ meats, in particular, are nutrient powerhouses, providing concentrated sources of vitamins A, D, E, K, B vitamins, and minerals like selenium and phosphorus. Including a variety of organ meats in the diet enhances nutrient density and supports metabolic processes.

Healing and Repair

Gut Lining Integrity

The amino acids and fats in animal products support gut lining integrity and repair. This is crucial for individuals with leaky gut syndrome or intestinal permeability issues, as it helps prevent undigested food particles and toxins from entering the bloodstream and causing immune reactions.

Reduced Inflammation

Inflammatory bowel conditions, such as Crohn's disease and ulcerative colitis, may benefit from the carnivore diet's anti-inflammatory properties. By reducing gut inflammation and supporting healing, the diet can alleviate symptoms and improve quality of life for those with chronic digestive disorders.

Practical Tips for Gut Health on the Carnivore Diet

Include Organ Meats: Organ meats like liver, kidney, and heart are rich in nutrients that support gut health, including vitamins, minerals, and amino acids. Start with small portions and gradually incorporate them into your meals.

Bone Broth: Homemade bone broth from animal bones and connective tissue provides collagen, gelatin, and essential minerals that support gut lining integrity and reduce inflammation.

Fatty Fish: Omega-3 fatty acids found in fatty fish like salmon and mackerel have anti-inflammatory properties that support gut health. Include these fish regularly in your diet for optimal omega-3 intake.

Monitor Hydration: Adequate hydration is essential for digestive health. Drink water throughout the day to support digestion and nutrient absorption.

Addressing Concerns

Fiber and Gut Health: The carnivore diet challenges conventional beliefs about fiber's role in gut health. While fiber may support microbial diversity in some individuals, the carnivore approach focuses on nutrient density and gut healing through animal products.

Adaptation Period: Recognize that the transition to a carnivore diet may involve an adaptation period for the gut microbiome. Monitor symptoms and consult with healthcare professionals as needed to optimize your dietary approach.

Nourish Your Gut with Animal Foods

The carnivore diet offers a unique perspective on gut health by emphasizing nutrient-dense animal products and minimizing potential gut irritants. By simplifying digestion, reducing inflammation, and supporting gut microbiome balance, the diet can provide relief for individuals with digestive disorders and promote overall well-being.

As you explore the carnivore lifestyle, prioritize nutrient density, personalized adaptation, and ongoing health assessments. Embrace the benefits of animal foods for gut health and discover how they can contribute to your journey towards optimal health and vitality. The following chapters will delve into practical strategies for meal planning, nutrient optimization, and sustainable practices on the carnivore diet. Nourish your gut, nourish your body, and thrive with a well-informed approach to carnivore nutrition.

CHAPTER 8: PHYSICAL PERFORMANCE ON A CARNIVORE DIET

Enhancing Strength, Endurance, and Recovery

The carnivore diet, centered around animal-based nutrition, offers unique advantages for physical performance. Whether you're an athlete, fitness enthusiast, or simply looking to improve your overall fitness levels, the carnivore diet provides a pathway to enhance strength, endurance, and recovery. In this chapter, we explore how animal products can optimize physical performance and support athletic goals.

Fueling Strength and Muscle Development

Protein Quality and Quantity

Animal products, such as beef, poultry, and seafood, are rich in high-quality proteins essential for muscle growth and repair. Protein intake is crucial for maintaining lean muscle mass and optimizing strength gains. The carnivore diet provides ample protein to support physical performance without the need for excessive carbohydrate consumption.

Amino Acid Profile

Meat contains all essential amino acids in optimal ratios for human nutrition. These amino acids are building blocks for muscle protein synthesis, promoting muscle recovery, and enhancing muscle strength. The bioavailability of amino acids in animal products ensures efficient utilization by the body during physical exertion.

Endurance and Energy Metabolism

Adaptation to Fat Metabolism

The carnivore diet promotes metabolic flexibility by shifting the body's primary fuel source from carbohydrates to fats. This adaptation, known as ketosis, enhances endurance by utilizing stored fat as a sustained energy source. Endurance athletes may benefit from improved fat oxidation rates and reduced reliance on glycogen stores during prolonged exercise.

Stable Energy Levels

Unlike carbohydrate-based diets that can lead to energy crashes, the carnivore diet provides a stable and consistent source of energy. Fat-rich animal products sustain energy levels throughout physical activity, supporting endurance and prolonged performance without fluctuations in blood sugar levels.

Recovery and Muscle Repair

Nutrient Density

Animal products, including organ meats and fatty fish, are nutrient-dense sources of vitamins, minerals, and antioxidants crucial for recovery and muscle repair. Nutrients like vitamin B12, iron, zinc, and omega-3 fatty acids support immune function, reduce inflammation, and enhance recovery processes post-exercise.

Anti-Inflammatory Benefits

The anti-inflammatory properties of animal fats and proteins can aid in reducing muscle soreness and inflammation following intense workouts. Omega-3 fatty acids found in fatty fish have been shown to accelerate muscle recovery and decrease oxidative stress associated with exercise-induced muscle damage.

Hormonal Balance and Performance

Testosterone Production

Dietary fats play a vital role in hormone production, including testosterone synthesis. The carnivore diet's emphasis on saturated and monounsaturated fats from animal sources supports optimal testosterone levels, which are essential for muscle growth, strength, and overall athletic performance.

Insulin Sensitivity

By reducing carbohydrate intake, the carnivore diet improves insulin sensitivity and promotes stable blood glucose levels. Enhanced insulin sensitivity facilitates nutrient uptake into muscle cells, supporting muscle glycogen replenishment and overall recovery post-exercise.

Practical Tips for Physical Performance on the Carnivore Diet

Pre-Workout Nutrition: Prioritize protein-rich meals before workouts to support muscle protein synthesis and energy levels. Include sources like beef, chicken, or eggs to provide essential amino acids and sustain performance.

Hydration: Maintain adequate hydration before, during, and after exercise to support muscle function, nutrient transport, and overall performance. Water, electrolyte-rich beverages, and bone broth can help replenish fluids and minerals lost during exercise.

Post-Workout Recovery: Consume a balanced meal containing protein and fats within the post-workout window to promote muscle repair and glycogen replenishment. Include nutrient-dense options such as steak, salmon, or organ meats for optimal recovery benefits.

Supplementation: Consider supplementing with creatine monohydrate to enhance muscle strength and power output during high-intensity exercise. Omega-3 fatty acids and vitamin D supplements may also support cardiovascular health and overall well-being.

Addressing Concerns

Carbohydrate Needs: While traditional sports nutrition emphasizes carbohydrates for energy, the carnivore diet demonstrates that fats can efficiently fuel physical performance. Adaptation to fat metabolism may require an adjustment period, but many athletes report sustained energy levels and improved endurance on a low-carb, high-fat diet.

Electrolyte Balance: Ensure adequate intake of sodium, potassium, and magnesium to support muscle function, hydration, and electrolyte balance during exercise. Incorporate electrolyte-rich foods like salted meats or electrolyte supplements as needed.

Thriving On Animal-Based Nutrition

The carnivore diet provides a unique approach to enhancing physical performance through nutrient-dense animal products and metabolic efficiency. By prioritizing protein quality, supporting endurance with fat metabolism, and optimizing recovery with nutrient-rich foods, individuals can achieve their athletic goals while maintaining overall health.

As you explore the carnivore lifestyle, tailor nutritional strategies to your specific fitness needs, monitor performance indicators, and consult with healthcare professionals or nutrition experts as necessary. Embrace the benefits of animal-based nutrition for strength, endurance, and recovery, and thrive on your journey towards peak physical performance and well-being.

In the upcoming chapters, we'll delve deeper into practical meal planning strategies, nutrient optimization tips, and sustainable practices to support your carnivore journey. Fuel your performance, embrace the power of animal foods, and excel in your athletic pursuits with informed dietary choices and holistic health approaches.

CHAPTER 9: MEAL PLANNING AND PREPARATION

Practical Tips for Everyday Carnivore Living

Embracing the carnivore diet involves more than just choosing animal-based foods—it requires thoughtful planning and preparation to ensure nutritional balance, variety, and enjoyment. In this chapter, we explore practical strategies for meal planning and preparation that support sustainable carnivore living and enhance your overall well-being.

Understanding Carnivore Nutrition

Focus on Animal Products

The foundation of the carnivore diet revolves around animal products such as beef, poultry, pork, lamb, fish, and organ meats. These foods provide essential nutrients like protein, healthy fats, vitamins, and minerals necessary for optimal health and performance.

Nutrient Density

Prioritize nutrient-dense cuts of meat and include a variety of animal sources to ensure a broad spectrum of nutrients. Organ meats, such as liver, kidney, and heart, are particularly rich in vitamins (A, D, E, K, B vitamins) and minerals (iron, zinc, selenium) that support various bodily functions.

Practical Meal Planning Tips

Weekly Meal Planning

Plan your meals ahead of time to streamline grocery shopping and ensure you have a variety of animal products on hand. Create a weekly menu that includes different cuts of meat, seafood, and organ meats to optimize nutrient intake and culinary diversity.

Balanced Macronutrients

Structure your meals to include a balance of protein and fats from animal sources. Adjust portion sizes based on your activity level, metabolic needs, and health goals. Protein intake should be sufficient to support muscle maintenance and repair, while fats provide sustained energy and satiety.

Incorporate Variety

Experiment with different cooking methods, seasonings, and cuts of meat to keep meals interesting and enjoyable. Incorporate seafood, eggs, and dairy (if tolerated) to expand your nutrient profile and culinary options while adhering to carnivore principles.

Practical Meal Preparation Tips

Batch Cooking

Prepare large batches of meat or meals that can be portioned and stored for future consumption. Use slow cookers, pressure cookers, or oven roasting methods to simplify cooking and maximize flavor. Batch cooking saves time and ensures you have nutritious meals readily available.

Include Organ Meats

Integrate organ meats into your diet to boost nutrient intake and support overall health. Experiment with recipes that incorporate liver, heart, or kidney for their unique flavors and nutritional benefits. Start with small portions and gradually increase consumption based on preference and tolerance.

Meal Timing and Frequency

Adapt meal timing and frequency to align with your lifestyle and metabolic needs. Some individuals thrive on two meals per day, while others prefer three meals or incorporate intermittent fasting. Listen to your body's hunger cues and adjust meal timing accordingly for optimal energy and satisfaction.

Practical Tips for Dining Out

Navigate Restaurant Menus

Choose restaurants that offer quality meat options and accommodate your dietary preferences. Opt for grilled or roasted meats without sauces, marinades, or breading. Customize orders to include additional fats or organ meats to enhance nutrient density.

Communication with Servers

Communicate your dietary needs clearly to restaurant staff to ensure your meal is prepared according to carnivore principles. Ask about ingredient lists, cooking methods, and modifications to meet your nutritional requirements and preferences.

Addressing Practical Challenges

Grocery Shopping

Select high-quality meat sources, including grass-fed beef, pasture-raised poultry, and wild-caught fish, when possible. Shop at local butcher shops or farmers' markets for fresh, sustainable options. Consider online suppliers for convenient delivery of specialty cuts or organ meats.

Budgeting Considerations

Prioritize nutrient-dense cuts of meat and plan meals based on seasonal availability and sales. Utilize cost-effective options like ground beef, chicken thighs, or pork shoulder for budget-friendly carnivore meals. Buy in bulk or freeze portions to maximize savings and minimize waste.

Embrace the Carnivore Lifestyle

Meal planning and preparation are essential components of successful carnivore living, ensuring nutrient adequacy, culinary enjoyment, and sustainable dietary practices. By focusing on animal-based nutrition, incorporating variety, and optimizing meal timing, you can thrive on the carnivore diet while supporting your health and wellness goals.

As you continue your carnivore journey, explore new recipes, experiment with different cuts of meat, and tailor your dietary approach to fit your individual needs. The following chapters will delve into nutrient optimization, sustainable practices, and lifestyle considerations to enhance your experience with the carnivore lifestyle. Embrace the simplicity and nutritional richness of animal foods, and discover the transformative power of carnivore living in your everyday life.

CHAPTER 10: CARNIVORE DIET FOR DIFFERENT LIFE STAGES

Adapting the Diet for Children, Adults, and Seniors

The carnivore diet, known for its simplicity and focus on animal-based nutrition, can be adapted to meet the unique nutritional needs and health considerations of individuals across different life stages. From childhood growth and development to adult health maintenance and senior vitality, this chapter explores how the carnivore diet can be tailored to support optimal nutrition and well-being throughout various stages of life.

Childhood Nutrition and Development

Nutrient-Dense Foundation

For children, the carnivore diet provides a nutrient-dense foundation that supports growth, development, and cognitive function. Animal products like beef, poultry, fish, and eggs supply essential proteins, fats, vitamins, and minerals necessary for bone health, muscle growth, and overall vitality.

Introducing Solid Foods

When introducing solid foods to infants, consider incorporating animal-based foods early on. Start with well-cooked and finely ground meats, egg yolks, and nutrient-rich organ meats to provide essential nutrients in a digestible form. Monitor tolerance and adjust textures as your child progresses.

Nutritional Adequacy

Ensure nutritional adequacy by including a variety of animal sources in your child's diet. Rotate between different cuts of meat, seafood options, and organ meats to optimize nutrient intake and support healthy development. Consult with pediatricians or nutrition experts for personalized guidance.

Adult Health and Longevity

Metabolic Efficiency

In adulthood, the carnivore diet promotes metabolic efficiency by reducing reliance on carbohydrates and optimizing fat metabolism. This metabolic flexibility supports weight management, insulin sensitivity, and sustained energy levels throughout the day.

Nutrient Optimization

Focus on nutrient-dense animal products to meet adult nutritional requirements. Incorporate a balance of proteins, fats, and micronutrients from sources like grass-fed beef, wild-caught fish, and organ meats. Tailor portion sizes and meal timing to individual activity levels and health goals.

Hormonal Balance

Animal fats and proteins support hormonal balance in adults, including testosterone production, which is essential for muscle maintenance, bone density, and overall vitality. Prioritize high-quality fats and proteins to support hormonal health and metabolic function.

Senior Health and Vitality

Nutritional Support

As individuals age, the carnivore diet provides essential nutrients that support senior health and vitality. Protein-rich foods aid in muscle maintenance and repair, while fats from animal sources contribute to cognitive function and cardiovascular health.

Bone Health

Include bone-in meats and collagen-rich foods like bone broth to support bone density and joint health. Nutrients such as calcium, phosphorus, and vitamin D found in animal products are crucial for maintaining skeletal integrity and reducing the risk of osteoporosis.

Digestive Comfort

The simplicity of the carnivore diet may benefit seniors by reducing digestive discomfort associated with high-fiber diets. Easily digestible animal proteins and fats support gastrointestinal health and nutrient absorption, promoting overall digestive comfort.

Practical Tips for Different Life Stages

Childhood:

- Introduce animal-based foods early and gradually to support nutrient absorption and digestive development.
- Monitor growth milestones and consult with healthcare providers for guidance on nutrient adequacy and dietary adjustments.

Adulthood:

- Prioritize nutrient density by including a variety of animal sources in your meals.
- Adjust protein and fat intake based on activity level, metabolic needs, and overall health goals.

Seniors:

- Include bone-in meats and collagen-rich foods to support bone health and joint function.
- Focus on nutrient absorption and digestive comfort by selecting easily digestible animal products.

Addressing Concerns

Nutrient Adequacy: Ensure comprehensive nutrient intake by varying animal sources and incorporating nutrient-dense options such as organ meats and seafood.

Digestive Health: Monitor digestive comfort and adjust dietary fiber intake based on individual tolerance and digestive needs.

Consultation: Consult with healthcare professionals or nutrition experts to personalize the carnivore diet according to individual health conditions, dietary preferences, and lifestyle factors.

Nourishing Wellness Across Generations

The carnivore diet offers a flexible approach to nutrition that can be adapted to meet the unique needs of children, adults, and seniors alike. By prioritizing nutrient density, metabolic efficiency, and digestive comfort, individuals can thrive on animal-based nutrition throughout different stages of life.

As you navigate the carnivore lifestyle, embrace the simplicity and nutritional richness of animal foods while tailoring dietary strategies to support optimal health and vitality. The following chapters will explore advanced topics in carnivore nutrition, sustainable practices, and holistic health considerations to empower your journey towards lifelong wellness. Nourish wellness across generations with the transformative power of the carnivore diet and discover its potential for sustained health and vitality throughout life's journey.

CHAPTER 11: ADDRESSING CHALLENGES

Overcoming Social, Psychological, And Practical Barriers

Embracing the carnivore diet presents unique challenges beyond nutritional considerations. From navigating social situations to overcoming psychological barriers and practical hurdles, this chapter explores strategies to successfully integrate and sustain the carnivore lifestyle amidst various challenges.

Social Challenges

Social Settings and Dining Out

Navigate social gatherings and dining out by communicating your dietary preferences respectfully. Choose restaurants that offer quality meat options and customize orders to align with carnivore principles. Focus on enjoying the company while making mindful food choices that support your health goals.

Family and Social Support

Educate family members and friends about the carnivore diet to foster understanding and support. Share information about the nutritional benefits and personal motivations behind your dietary choices. Collaborate on meal planning or hosting events that accommodate your preferences without compromising social interactions.

Psychological Barriers

Mindset and Motivation

Maintain a positive mindset and motivation by focusing on the benefits of the carnivore diet for your health and well-being. Reflect on personal progress, improvements in energy levels, mental clarity, or physical performance as motivating factors. Seek support from online communities or peer groups sharing similar dietary journeys.

Emotional Eating and Cravings

Address emotional eating triggers and cravings by identifying alternative coping strategies. Practice mindfulness techniques, engage in physical activity, or explore creative outlets to manage stress and emotions effectively. Emphasize nutrient-dense meals that satisfy hunger and support emotional balance without relying on carbohydrate-rich foods.

Practical Hurdles

Grocery Shopping and Meal Preparation

Optimize grocery shopping by selecting high-quality meat sources, including grass-fed beef, pasture-raised poultry, and wild-caught fish. Plan meals ahead of time to streamline shopping trips and ensure variety in your carnivore diet. Utilize online suppliers or local butcher shops for specialty cuts or organ meats.

Budgeting and Cost Considerations

Manage budgeting and cost considerations by prioritizing nutrient-dense cuts of meat and seasonal options. Buy in bulk or freeze portions to maximize savings and minimize waste. Explore cost-effective options like ground beef, chicken thighs, or organ meats for affordable carnivore meals without compromising nutritional quality.

Long-Term Sustainability

Adaptation and Flexibility

Adapt the carnivore diet to align with long-term sustainability and individual health goals. Consider occasional deviations or modifications based on personal preferences, seasonal availability, or social occasions. Focus on nutrient density, metabolic health, and overall well-being while maintaining flexibility within the carnivore framework.

Health Monitoring and Support

Monitor health markers, including blood lipids, nutrient levels, and overall well-being, to assess the impact of the carnivore diet on your health. Consult healthcare professionals or nutrition experts for guidance on optimizing nutrient intake, addressing concerns, and maintaining balanced nutrition throughout your carnivore journey.

Addressing Concerns

Social Integration: Develop strategies to navigate social settings and dining out while adhering to carnivore principles. Communicate dietary preferences respectfully and seek supportive environments that accommodate your health goals.

Psychological Resilience: Cultivate psychological resilience by focusing on positive outcomes and personal motivations for adopting the carnivore diet. Manage emotional eating triggers and cravings with effective coping strategies and support systems.

Practical Solutions: Implement practical solutions for grocery shopping, meal preparation, and budgeting to sustain the carnivore lifestyle effectively. Prioritize nutrient-dense options and adapt dietary practices to fit your lifestyle and long-term health objectives.

Embrace Resilience and Adaptability

Overcoming challenges associated with the carnivore diet requires resilience, adaptability, and a commitment to prioritizing health and well-being. By addressing social, psychological, and practical barriers with informed strategies and support systems, individuals can sustainably integrate and thrive on animal-based nutrition.

As you navigate the carnivore lifestyle, embrace opportunities for growth, learning, and personal empowerment. The following chapters will explore advanced topics in carnivore nutrition, lifestyle optimization, and holistic health considerations to support your journey towards sustained vitality and well-being. Embrace resilience, overcome challenges, and thrive on the transformative power of the carnivore diet in enhancing your quality of life.

CHAPTER 12: SUCCESS STORIES

Real-Life Transformations And Testimonials

The carnivore diet has garnered attention for its potential to transform lives through improved health, vitality, and well-being. In this chapter, we explore real-life success stories and testimonials from individuals who have embraced the carnivore lifestyle, sharing their journeys of transformation, health improvements, and personal triumphs.

Personal Testimonials

Weight Loss and Body Composition

Many individuals have experienced significant weight loss and improvements in body composition on the carnivore diet. By focusing on nutrient-dense animal products and eliminating carbohydrates, they have achieved sustainable weight management and reduced body fat percentage.

Mental Clarity and Cognitive Function

Carnivore enthusiasts often report enhanced mental clarity, focus, and cognitive function. By minimizing dietary inflammation and stabilizing blood sugar levels, they experience improved concentration, memory retention, and overall mental well-being.

Energy Levels and Physical Performance

Individuals following the carnivore diet frequently cite increased energy levels and enhanced physical performance. By optimizing fat metabolism and supporting muscle recovery with animal proteins, they achieve peak athletic performance and sustained endurance.

Health Improvements

Digestive Health

Many carnivore adopters have found relief from digestive disorders such as irritable bowel syndrome (IBS) and acid reflux. By eliminating potential irritants and focusing on easily digestible animal foods, they experience reduced bloating, gas, and gastrointestinal discomfort.

Autoimmune Conditions

Some individuals with autoimmune conditions, such as rheumatoid arthritis and psoriasis, have reported symptom relief and disease management on the carnivore diet. By reducing inflammatory triggers and supporting immune function with nutrient-dense meats, they achieve greater symptom control and improved quality of life.

Hormonal Balance and Metabolic Health

Balancing hormones and improving metabolic health are common benefits noted by those on the carnivore diet. By optimizing insulin sensitivity and supporting hormone production with animal fats and proteins, they manage conditions like PCOS (polycystic ovary syndrome) and achieve hormonal equilibrium.

Lifestyle Transformations

Emotional Well-Being

Beyond physical health benefits, individuals often highlight improvements in emotional well-being and mood stability on the carnivore diet. By regulating neurotransmitters and supporting brain health with animal-based nutrition, they experience reduced anxiety, depression, and stress levels.

Sleep Quality

Enhanced sleep quality is frequently reported among carnivore practitioners. By stabilizing blood sugar levels and promoting relaxation with nutrient-dense meals, they achieve deeper, more restorative sleep patterns and wake up feeling refreshed.

Inspirational Journeys

Personal Growth and Empowerment

Through their carnivore journeys, many individuals experience personal growth, empowerment, and a renewed sense of control over their health and well-being. By embracing dietary changes and prioritizing self-care, they inspire others to explore alternative approaches to health and vitality.

Community Support and Connection

Engaging with the carnivore community provides valuable support, encouragement, and camaraderie. By sharing experiences, exchanging recipes, and celebrating milestones, individuals foster a sense of belonging and collective empowerment in their dietary choices.

Celebrating Transformative Journeys

The success stories and testimonials of individuals on the carnivore diet underscore its potential to transform lives through improved health outcomes, vitality, and holistic well-being. By embracing nutrient-dense animal foods and prioritizing personal health goals, individuals inspire others to explore the transformative power of the carnivore lifestyle.

As you embark on your own carnivore journey, draw inspiration from these real-life transformations and testimonials. Explore the benefits of animal-based nutrition, prioritize holistic health, and celebrate your progress towards optimal well-being. The following chapters will delve into advanced topics, practical strategies, and holistic approaches to support your continued success on the carnivore diet. Embrace your journey, celebrate your achievements, and thrive with the empowering benefits of the carnivore lifestyle.

CHAPTER 13: ADVANCED CARNIVORE TECHNIQUES

Incorporating Fasting, Organ Meats, and More

The carnivore diet offers flexibility and customization through advanced techniques that optimize nutritional intake, support metabolic health, and enhance overall well-being. In this chapter, we explore advanced strategies such as fasting protocols, integration of nutrient-dense organ meats, and additional practices to elevate your carnivore experience.

Intermittent Fasting and Extended Fasting

Metabolic Benefits

Incorporating intermittent fasting (IF) or extended fasting can amplify the benefits of the carnivore diet. By alternating periods of eating with periods of fasting, you enhance metabolic flexibility, promote autophagy (cellular repair process), and optimize fat metabolism for sustained energy and weight management.

Fasting Protocols

Experiment with fasting protocols that suit your lifestyle and goals. Popular approaches include:

- 16/8 Method: Daily fasting for 16 hours with an 8-hour eating window.
- OMAD (One Meal a Day): Consuming all daily calories within a single meal.
- Alternate Day Fasting: Cycling between days of normal eating and fasting days.

Guidelines and Adaptation

Start with shorter fasting durations and gradually increase fasting periods based on individual tolerance and metabolic adaptation. Stay hydrated, prioritize electrolyte balance, and monitor hunger cues to ensure safe and effective fasting practices on the carnivore diet.

Nutrient-Dense Organ Meats

Health Benefits

Integrate nutrient-dense organ meats into your carnivore diet to enhance nutrient variety and support optimal health. Organ meats, such as liver, heart, kidney, and brain, are rich in vitamins (A, D, E, K, B vitamins) and minerals (iron, zinc, selenium) crucial for immune function, energy metabolism, and overall vitality.

Preparation and Incorporation

Experiment with recipes that incorporate organ meats to diversify your nutrient intake and culinary experience. Start with small portions and gradually increase consumption based on taste preferences and tolerance. Consider blending or grinding organ meats into ground beef or patties for convenient preparation.

Bone Broth and Collagen

Joint and Gut Health

Bone broth is a valuable addition to the carnivore diet, providing collagen, gelatin, and essential amino acids that support joint health, gut integrity, and skin elasticity. Regular consumption of bone broth promotes digestive comfort, reduces inflammation, and enhances nutrient absorption.

Homemade Preparation

Prepare homemade bone broth using grass-fed beef bones, chicken carcasses, or pork bones. Simmer bones in water with vegetables and herbs for several hours to extract beneficial nutrients and flavors. Store broth in batches for convenient use in soups, stews, or as a standalone beverage.

Fermented Foods and Probiotics

Digestive Support

Incorporate fermented foods like sauerkraut, kimchi, or fermented dairy (if tolerated) to enhance gut health and support digestive function on the carnivore diet. Fermented foods contain beneficial probiotic bacteria that promote microbial diversity, immune function, and nutrient absorption.

Quality and Selection

Choose fermented foods with minimal additives and low sugar content to align with carnivore principles. Experiment with homemade fermentation or select commercially available options that prioritize natural ingredients and traditional preparation methods.

Practical Implementation Tips

Gradual Integration

Introduce advanced techniques, such as fasting protocols or organ meats, gradually to allow for adaptation and enjoyment. Monitor how your body responds to changes in dietary practices and adjust accordingly based on personal preferences and health goals.

Consultation and Guidance

Consult with healthcare professionals or nutrition experts for personalized advice on integrating advanced carnivore techniques into your dietary regimen. Discuss any underlying health conditions, nutrient requirements, or metabolic considerations to optimize your carnivore experience.

Elevating Your Carnivore Journey

Advanced carnivore techniques empower individuals to customize their dietary approach, optimize nutrient intake, and enhance overall well-being through strategic practices like fasting, organ meat consumption, and fermented foods. By embracing these advanced strategies, you can elevate your carnivore journey, support metabolic health, and achieve sustainable wellness.

As you explore the benefits of fasting, nutrient-dense organ meats, and other advanced techniques, prioritize balance, adaptation, and personalized wellness goals. The following chapters will delve into lifestyle optimization, sustainable practices, and holistic health considerations to support your continued success on the carnivore diet. Elevate your journey, embrace nutritional richness, and thrive with the empowering benefits of advanced carnivore techniques in enhancing your quality of life.

CHAPTER 14: INTEGRATING CARNIVORE WITH MODERN LIFE

Balancing Tradition And Convenience

Integrating the carnivore diet into modern lifestyles requires balancing traditional dietary principles with practical considerations for convenience, social dynamics, and sustainability. In this chapter, we explore strategies to seamlessly incorporate carnivore principles into contemporary living while honoring nutritional integrity and personal health goals.

Embracing Carnivore Principles

Nutrient-Dense Focus

Prioritize nutrient-dense animal products, including beef, poultry, fish, and organ meats, to support optimal health and well-being on the carnivore diet. Choose high-quality sources such as grass-fed beef, pasture-raised poultry, and wild-caught fish whenever possible to enhance nutritional value.

Simplicity and Minimalism

Simplify meal preparation by focusing on whole animal foods and minimal ingredients. Embrace the simplicity of carnivore meals while maximizing nutritional richness and culinary satisfaction. Experiment with different cuts of meat, cooking methods, and seasonings to diversify your palate and meal variety.

Practical Tips for Modern Living

Meal Planning and Batch Cooking

Plan meals in advance to streamline grocery shopping and ensure dietary adherence. Batch cooking allows for efficient preparation of carnivore meals that can be portioned and stored for convenience throughout the week. Use slow cookers, pressure cookers, or meal prep techniques to optimize time management.

On-the-Go Options

Prepare portable carnivore snacks or meals for busy schedules or travel. Pack sliced meats, hard-boiled eggs, or jerky made from quality animal sources to maintain nutritional balance and sustain energy levels while on the move. Explore carnivore-friendly restaurants or fast food options that align with your dietary preferences.

Social And Dining Considerations

Navigating Social Settings

Communicate your dietary preferences respectfully in social settings while prioritizing health goals. Choose restaurants that offer quality meat options and customize orders to meet carnivore principles. Focus on enjoying the company and social interactions while making mindful food choices.

Family and Meal Preparation

Involve family members in meal planning and preparation to foster understanding and support for carnivore dietary practices. Collaborate on recipes that accommodate both carnivore and non-carnivore preferences to promote inclusivity and shared dining experiences.

Technology and Resources

Online Communities and Support

Engage with online carnivore communities to share experiences, exchange recipes, and seek support from like-minded individuals. Utilize social media platforms, forums, or dedicated carnivore websites to access resources, research, and motivational content that enhance your carnivore journey.

Nutritional Tracking and Tools

Utilize nutritional tracking apps or tools to monitor dietary intake and ensure nutrient adequacy on the carnivore diet. Track protein, fat, and micronutrient consumption to optimize health outcomes and adjust meal planning based on individual needs and goals.

Sustainability and Long-Term Adherence

Environmental Impact

Consider sustainability factors when choosing animal products for the carnivore diet. Select locally sourced or sustainably raised meats to minimize environmental footprint and support ethical farming practices. Explore regenerative agriculture practices that prioritize soil health and ecosystem restoration.

Flexibility and Adaptation

Maintain flexibility within the carnivore framework to accommodate lifestyle changes, seasonal availability, or social occasions. Adapt meal planning and dietary practices based on personal preferences, health considerations, and evolving nutritional goals for long-term adherence and sustainability.

Embrace Modern Carnivore Living

Integrating the carnivore diet with modern life requires a balance of tradition, convenience, and nutritional integrity. By embracing carnivore principles while navigating practical challenges and social dynamics, individuals can optimize health, well-being, and dietary satisfaction in contemporary lifestyles.

As you embark on your carnivore journey, prioritize simplicity, nutritional richness, and personalized wellness goals. The following chapters will explore advanced topics, holistic health considerations, and lifestyle optimization strategies to support your continued success and fulfillment on the carnivore diet. Embrace modern carnivore living, celebrate dietary empowerment, and thrive with the transformative benefits of animal-based nutrition in enhancing your quality of life.

CHAPTER 15: THE FUTURE OF NUTRITION

How The Carnivore Diet Is Shaping Health Trends

The carnivore diet has emerged as a provocative approach to nutrition, challenging conventional dietary norms and reshaping perspectives on health and wellness. In this final chapter, we explore the evolving landscape of nutrition and the significant impact of the carnivore diet on current health trends and future possibilities.

Reevaluating Dietary Paradigms

Shift in Nutritional Paradigms

The carnivore diet represents a shift away from traditional dietary recommendations that emphasize plant-based foods and grains. By focusing on animal-based nutrition, it challenges prevailing beliefs about dietary diversity and optimal nutrient sources for human health.

Scientific Inquiry and Exploration

Growing interest in the carnivore diet has sparked scientific inquiry and exploration into its potential benefits and implications for health outcomes. Research initiatives are investigating metabolic responses, nutrient bioavailability, and long-term health effects to expand understanding and evidence-based practice.

Health Benefits and Therapeutic Potential

Metabolic Health and Weight Management

Advocates of the carnivore diet highlight its potential benefits for metabolic health, including improved insulin sensitivity, reduced inflammation, and enhanced fat metabolism. By minimizing carbohydrate intake and prioritizing animal fats and proteins, individuals may achieve sustainable weight management and metabolic resilience.

Autoimmune Conditions and Inflammatory Disorders

Some studies suggest that the carnivore diet may benefit individuals with autoimmune conditions or inflammatory disorders. By eliminating potential dietary triggers and supporting immune function with nutrient-dense animal foods, individuals may experience symptom relief and disease management.

Sustainability and Environmental Considerations

Ecological Footprint

Critics raise concerns about the environmental impact of animal-based diets like carnivore, citing resource consumption and greenhouse gas emissions associated with meat production. Advocates argue for sustainable farming practices and regenerative agriculture initiatives that prioritize soil health and ecosystem restoration.

Ethical Considerations

Ethical considerations surrounding animal welfare and farming practices are central to discussions about the carnivore diet. Advocates emphasize the importance of humane treatment and ethical sourcing of animal products to align with principles of compassion and sustainability.

Cultural and Societal Impact

Cultural Perspectives and Dietary Traditions

The carnivore diet prompts reflection on cultural perspectives and dietary traditions worldwide. It challenges cultural norms regarding food diversity and culinary practices while fostering dialogue about personalized nutrition and ancestral eating patterns.

Social Influence and Lifestyle Choices

Social media platforms, celebrity endorsements, and online communities play a significant role in shaping perceptions and adoption of the carnivore diet. Advocates share success stories, recipes, and motivational content that inspire others to explore alternative approaches to health and dietary empowerment.

Looking Ahead: Future Directions

Research Advancements

Future research is anticipated to explore the long-term effects of the carnivore diet on health outcomes, including cardiovascular health, gut microbiome diversity, and aging processes. Scientific advancements will contribute to evidence-based recommendations and personalized dietary guidelines.

Integration with Technology

Advancements in nutritional tracking apps, genetic testing, and personalized medicine will facilitate individualized approaches to carnivore nutrition. Technology integration will empower individuals to optimize nutrient intake, monitor health metrics, and achieve personalized wellness goals.

Embracing Evolutionary Perspectives

The carnivore diet represents a dynamic evolution in nutrition, challenging conventional wisdom and inspiring innovation in health and wellness. By exploring its impact on health trends, environmental considerations, and societal perspectives, individuals can make informed choices that align with their health goals and ethical values.

As you reflect on the future of nutrition and the transformative potential of the carnivore diet, embrace opportunities for growth, discovery, and holistic well-being. The journey towards optimal health is shaped by ongoing exploration, scientific inquiry, and individual empowerment. Celebrate the evolution of nutrition, embrace ancestral wisdom, and thrive with the empowering benefits of the carnivore diet in enhancing your quality of life and well-being.

CONCLUSION: EMBRACING THE CARNIVORE REVOLUTION FOR LIFELONG HEALTH

The carnivore diet represents more than just a dietary approach—it embodies a revolutionary shift in how we perceive nutrition, health, and well-being. As we conclude this exploration into the carnivore lifestyle, it becomes clear that embracing this dietary revolution offers profound implications for lifelong health and vitality.

Reflecting on Nutritional Evolution

Throughout this journey, we've delved into the ancestral roots of human nutrition, explored the scientific underpinnings of the carnivore diet, and examined its practical applications across different life stages. From understanding the metabolic benefits of animal-based nutrition to addressing common misconceptions and navigating social challenges, each chapter has illuminated the transformative potential of the carnivore lifestyle.

Empowering Personal Health

Embracing the carnivore diet empowers individuals to reclaim control over their health by prioritizing nutrient-dense animal foods and minimizing reliance on processed carbohydrates and plant-based foods. By optimizing metabolic health, supporting digestive comfort, and enhancing mental clarity, the carnivore diet offers a pathway to sustainable wellness and vitality.

Navigating Challenges with Resilience

Challenges such as social integration, psychological barriers, and practical hurdles are inherent to adopting any dietary change, including carnivore. However, with resilience, adaptability, and support from communities and healthcare professionals, individuals can navigate these challenges and sustainably integrate carnivore principles into modern lifestyles.

Celebrating Transformative Journeys

The success stories and testimonials shared throughout this exploration underscore the profound impact of the carnivore diet on individuals' lives. From weight loss and improved physical performance to enhanced emotional well-being and disease management, these journeys inspire others to explore alternative approaches to health and dietary empowerment.

Embracing the Future of Nutrition

Looking forward, the carnivore diet continues to shape health trends, challenge dietary norms, and inspire ongoing research into its potential benefits and implications. As advancements in science, technology, and sustainability converge, individuals have unprecedented opportunities to personalize their nutritional approach and optimize health outcomes.

Call to Action: Thriving with Carnivore Nutrition

As you embark on your carnivore journey or contemplate its potential benefits, I encourage you to embrace ancestral wisdom, scientific inquiry, and personal empowerment. Explore the transformative power of the carnivore diet, celebrate your progress and achievements, and prioritize holistic well-being in your pursuit of lifelong health.

Whether you are beginning your carnivore journey, navigating challenges along the way, or advocating for broader acceptance and understanding, remember that each step contributes to a larger movement towards health, vitality, and personal empowerment.

Embrace the Carnivore Diet Revolution

In conclusion, the carnivore diet offers a revolutionary paradigm for enhancing health, vitality, and quality of life. By embracing nutrient-dense animal foods and honoring evolutionary perspectives on human nutrition, individuals can cultivate resilience, achieve optimal wellness, and thrive in today's dynamic world.

Thank you for joining me on this journey into the carnivore revolution. May your pursuit of lifelong health be guided by knowledge, supported by community, and enriched by the transformative benefits of the carnivore lifestyle.